The Vibrant Dash Diet Recipe Book

Healthy And Easy Dash Diet Recipes For Weight Loss

Peter Haley

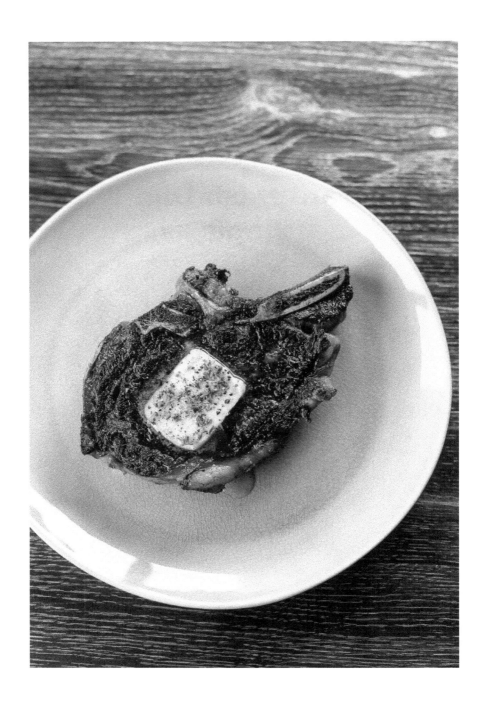

Table of contents

Salmon in Dill Sauce

Prep Time: 10 mins

Servings: 6

Cooking: 1 hours and 30 mins

Ingredients:

- 6 salmon fillets
- 1 cup low-fat, low-sodium chicken broth
- 1 tsp. cayenne pepper
- 2 tbsp Fresh lemon juice
- 2 cup water
- ¼ cup chopped fresh dill

Directions:

1. In a slow cooker, mix together water, broth, lemon juice, lemon juice and dill.
2. Arrange salmon fillets on top, skin side down.
3. Sprinkle with cayenne pepper.
4. Set the slow cooker on low.

5. Cover and cook for about 1-2 hours.

Nutrition:

- Calories 360
- Fat 8 g
- Carbs 44 g
- Protein 28 g

Salmon and Potatoes Mix

Prep Time: 10 mins

Servings: 4

Cooking: 3-4 mins

Ingredients:

- 4 oz. chopped smoked salmon
- 1 tbsp essential olive oil
- Black pepper
- 1 tbsp chopped chives
- ¼ cup coconut cream
- 1 ½ lbs. chopped potatoes
- 2 tsps. Prepared horseradish

Directions:

1. Heat up a pan using the oil over medium heat, add potatoes and cook for 10 mins.

2. Add salmon, chives, horseradish, cream and black pepper, toss, cook for 1 minute more, divide between plates and serve.

Nutrition:

- Calories 233
- Fat 6 g
- Carbs 9 g
- Protein 11 g

Roasted Hake

Prep Time: 20 mins

Servings: 4

Cooking: 3-4 mins

Ingredients:

- ½ cup tomato sauce
- 2 sliced tomatoes
- Fresh parsley
- ½ cup grated cheese
- 4 lbs. deboned hake fish

Directions:

1. Season the fish with salt. Pan-fry the fish until half-done.
2. Shape foil into containers according to the number of fish pieces.

3. Pour tomato sauce into each foil dish; arrange the fish, then the tomato slices, again add tomato sauce and sprinkle with grated cheese.
4. Bake in the oven at 400 F until there is a golden crust.
5. Serve with fresh parsley.

Nutrition:

- Calories 421
- Fat 48.7 g
- Carbs 2.4 g
- Protein 17.4 g

Sautéed Fish Fillets

Prep Time: 5 mins

Servings: 4

Cooking: 3-4 mins

Ingredients:

- 1 tbsp extra-virgin olive oil
- 1 lb. sliced haddock
- 1/3 cup all-purpose flour
- Freshly ground pepper

Directions:

1. Combine flour, salt and pepper in a shallow dish; thoroughly dredge fillets
2. Heat oil in a large nonstick skillet over medium-high heat.
3. Add the fish, working in batches if necessary, and cook until lightly browned and just opaque in the center, 3 to 4 mins per side.

4. Serve immediately.

Nutrition:

- Calories 111
- Fat 11 g
- Carbs 15 g
- Protein 13 g

Coconut Cream Shrimp

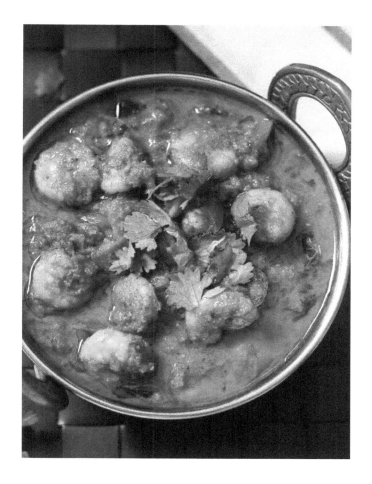

Prep Time: 10 mins

Servings: 2

Ingredients:

- 1 tbsp coconut cream
- ½ tsp. lime juice
- ¼ tsp. black pepper
- 1 tbsp parsley
- 1 lb. cooked, peeled and deveined shrimp
- ¼ tsp. chopped jalapeno

Directions:

In a bowl, mix the shrimp while using cream, jalapeno, lime juice, parsley and black pepper, toss, divide into small bowls and serve.

Nutrition:

- Calories 183
- Fat 5 g
- Carbs 12 g
- Protein 8 g

Cinnamon Salmon

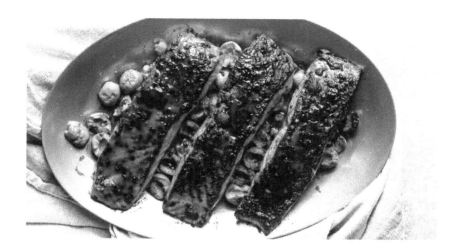

Prep Time: 10 mins

Servings: 2

Ingredients:

- 1 tbsp organic essential olive oil
- Black pepper
- 1 tbsp cinnamon powder
- 2 de-boned salmon fillets

Directions:

1. Heat up a pan with the oil over medium heat, add pepper and cinnamon and stir well.
2. Add salmon, skin side up, cook for 5 mins on both sides, divide between plates and serve by using a side salad.

Nutrition:

- Calories 220
- Fat 8 g
- Carbs 11 g
- Protein 8 g

Scallops and Strawberry Mix

Prep Time: 20 mins

Servings: 2

Ingredients:

- 1 tbsp lime juice
- ½ cup Pico de gallo
- Black pepper
- 4 oz. scallops
- ½ cup chopped strawberries

Directions:

1. Heat up a pan over medium heat, add scallops, cook for 3 mins on both sides and take away heat,
2. In a bowl, mix strawberries with lime juice, Pico de gallo, scallops and pepper, toss and serve cold.

Nutrition:

- Calories 169
- Fat 2 g
- Carbs 8 g
- Protein 13 g

Cod Peas Relish

Prep Time: 18-20 mins

Servings: 4-5

Cooking: 5 mins

Ingredients:

- 1 cup peas
- 2 tbsp Capers
- 4 de-boned medium cod fillets
- 3 tbsp Olive oil
- ¼ tsp. black pepper
- 2 tbsp Lime juice
- 2 tbsp Chopped shallots
- 1 ½ tbsp Chopped oregano

Directions:

1. Heat up 1 tbsp olive oil in a saucepan over medium flame
2. Add the fillets, cook for 5 mins on each side; set aside.

3. In a bowl of large size, thoroughly mix the oregano, shallots, lime juice, peas, capers, black pepper, and 2 tbsp olive oil.
4. Toss and serve with the cooked fish.

Nutrition:

- Calories 224
- Fat 11 g
- Carbs 7 g
- Protein 24 g

Baked Haddock

Prep Time: 10 mins

Servings: 4

Cooking: 35 mins

Ingredients:

- 1 tsp. chopped dill
- 3 tsps. Water
- Cooking spray
- 1 lb. chopped haddock
- 2 tbsp Fresh lemon juice
- 2 tbsp Avocado mayonnaise

Directions:

1. Spray a baking dish with a few oil, add fish, water, freshly squeezed lemon juice, salt, black pepper, mayo and dill, toss, introduce inside the oven and bake at 350 º F for the half-hour.
2. Divide between plates and serve.

Nutrition:

- Calories 264
- Fat 4 g
- Carbs 7 g
- Protein 12 g

Hot Tuna Steak

Prep Time: 10 mins

Servings: 6

Ingredients:

- 2 tbsp Fresh lemon juice
- Roasted orange garlic mayonnaise
- ¼ cup whole black peppercorns
- 6 sliced tuna steaks
- 2 tbsp Extra-virgin olive oil

Directions:

1. Place the tuna in a bowl to fit. Add the oil, lemon juice, salt and pepper. Turn the tuna to coat well in the marinade. Let rest 15 to 20 mins, turning once.
2. Place the peppercorns in a double thickness of plastic bags. Tap the peppercorns with a heavy saucepan or small mallet to crush them coarsely. Place on a large plate.
3. When ready to cook the tuna, dip the edges into the crushed peppercorns. Heat a nonstick skillet over

medium heat. Sear the tuna steaks, in batches if necessary, for 4 mins per side for medium-rare fish, adding 2 to 3 tbsps of the marinade to the skillet if necessary to prevent sticking.

4. Serve dolloped with roasted orange garlic mayonnaise

Nutrition:

- Calories 124
- Fat 0.4 g
- Carbs 0.6 g
- Protein 28 g

Marinated Fish Steaks

Prep Time: 10 mins

Servings: 4

Cooking: 12 mins

Ingredients:

- 4 lime wedges
- 2 tbsp Lime juice
- 2 minced garlic cloves
- 2 tsps. Olive oil
- 1 tbsp snipped fresh oregano
- 1 lb. fresh swordfish
- 1 tsp. lemon-pepper seasoning

Directions:

1. Rinse fish steaks; pat dry with paper towels. Cut into four serving size pieces, if necessary.

2. In a shallow dish combine lime juice, oregano, oil, lemon-pepper seasoning, and garlicup Add fish; turn to coat with marinade.
3. Cover and marinate in refrigerator for 30 mins to 1-1/2 hours, turning steaks occasionally. Drain fish, reserving marinade.
4. Place fish on the greased unheated rack of a broiler pan.
5. Broil 4 inches from the heat for 8 to 12 mins or until fish begins to flake when tested with a fork, turning once and brushing with reserved marinade halfway through cooking. Discard any remaining marinade.
6. Before serving, squeeze the juice from one lime wedge over each steak.

Nutrition:

- Calories 240
- Fat 6 g
- Carbs 19 g
- Protein 12 g

Baked Tomato Hake

Prep Time: 35-40 mins

Servings: 4-5

Ingredients:

- ½ cup tomato sauce
- 1 tbsp olive oil
- Parsley
- 2 sliced tomatoes
- ½ cup grated cheese
- 4 lbs. de-boned and sliced hake fish

Directions:

1. Preheat the oven to 400 º F.
2. Season the fish with salt.
3. In a skillet or saucepan; stir-fry the fish in the olive oil until half-done.
4. Take four foil papers to cover the fish.
5. Shape the foil to resemble containers; add the tomato sauce into each foil container.
6. Add the fish, tomato slices, and top with grated cheese.

7. Bake until you get a golden crust, for approximately 20-25 mins.
8. Open the packs and top with parsley.

Nutrition:

- Calories 265
- Fat 15 g
- Carbs 18 g
- Protein 22 g

Cheesy Tuna Pasta

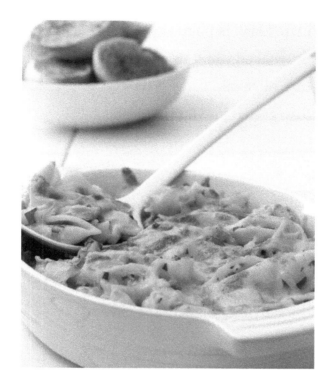

Prep Time: 5-8 min

Servings: 3-4

Ingredients:

- 2 cup arugula
- ¼ cup chopped green onions

- 1 tbs. red vinegar
- 5 oz. drained canned tuna
- ¼ tsp. black pepper
- 2 oz. cooked whole-wheat pasta
- 1 tbsp olive oil
- 1 tbsp grated low-fat parmesan

Directions:

1. Cook the pasta in unsalted water until ready. Drain and set aside.
2. In a bowl of large size, thoroughly mix the tuna, green onions, vinegar, oil, arugula, pasta, and black pepper.
3. Toss well and top with the cheese.

Nutrition:

- Calories 566.3
- Fat 42.4 g
- Carbs 18.6 g
- Protein 29.8 g

Herb-Coated Baked Cod with Honey

Prep Time: 5 mins

Servings: 2

Cooking: 10 mins

Ingredients:

- 6 tbsp Herb-flavored stuffing
- 8 oz. cod fillets
- 2 tbsp Honey

Directions:

1. Preheat your oven to 375 º F.
2. Spray a baking pan lightly with cooking spray.
3. Put the herb-flavored stuffing in a bag and close. Squash the stuffing until it gets crumbly.
4. Coat the fishes with honey and get rid of the remaining honey. Add one fillet to the bag of stuffing and shake gently to coat the fish completely.

5. Transfer the cod to the baking pan and repeat the process for the second fish.
6. Wrap the fillets with foil and bake until firm and opaque all through when you test with the tip of a knife blade, about ten mins.
7. Serve hot.

Nutrition:

- Calories 185
- Fat 1 g
- Carbs 23 g
- Protein 21 g

Tender Salmon in Mustard Sauce

Prep Time: 10 mins

Servings: 2

Cooking: 20 mins

Ingredients:

- 5 tbsp Minced dill
- 2/3 cup sour cream
- 2 tbsp Dijon mustard
- 1 tsp. garlic powder
- 5 oz. salmon fillets
- 2-3 tbsp Lemon juice

Directions:

1. Mix sour cream, mustard, lemon juice and dill.
2. Season the fillets with pepper and garlic powder.
3. Arrange the salmon on a baking sheet skin side down and cover with the prepared mustard sauce.
4. Bake for 20 mins at 390°F.

Nutrition:

- Calories 318
- Fat 12 g
- Carbs 8 g
- Protein 40.9 g

Broiled White Sea Bass

Prep Time: 5 mins

Servings: 2

Cooking: 10 mins

Ingredients:

- 1 tsp. minced garlic
- 1 tbsp lemon juice
- 8 oz. white sea bass fillets
- ¼ tsp. salt-free herbed seasoning blend

Directions:

1. Preheat the broiler and position the rack 4 inches from the heat source.
2. Lightly spray a baking pan with cooking spray. Place the fillets in the pan. Sprinkle the lemon juice, garlic, herbed seasoning and pepper over the fillets.
3. Broil until the fish is opaque throughout when tested with a tip of a knife, about 8 to 10 mins.

Nutrition:

- Calories 114
- Fat 2 g
- Carbs 2 g
- Protein 21 g

Tuna and Shallots

Prep Time: 10 mins

Servings: 4

Cooking: 10 mins

Ingredients:

- ½ cup low-sodium chicken stock
- 1 tbsp olive oil
- 4 boneless and skinless tuna fillets
- 2 chopped shallots
- 1 tsp. sweet paprika
- 2 tbsp lime juice

Directions:

1. Heat up a pan with the oil over medium-high heat, add shallots and sauté for 3 mins.
2. Add the fish and cook it for 4 mins on each side.
3. Add the rest of the ingredients, cook everything for 3 mins more, divide between plates and serve.

Nutrition:

- Calories 404
- Fat 34.6 g
- Carbs 3 g
- Protein 21.4 g

Paprika Tuna

Prep Time: 4 mins

Servings: 4

Cooking: 5 mins

Ingredients:

- ½ tsp. chili powder
- 2 tsps. sweet paprika
- ¼ tsp. black pepper
- 2 tbsp olive oil
- 4 boneless tuna steaks

Directions:

Heat up a pan with the oil over medium-high heat, add the tuna steaks, season with paprika, black pepper and chili powder, cook for 5 mins on each side, divide between plates and serve with a side salad.

Nutrition:

- Calories 455
- Fat 20.6 g
- Carbs 0.8 g
- Protein 63.8 g

Ginger Sea Bass Mix

Prep Time: 10 mins

Servings: 4

Cooking: 10 mins

Ingredients:

- 4 boneless sea bass fillets
- 2 tbsp olive oil
- 1 tsp. grated ginger
- 1 tbsp chopped cilantro
- Black pepper
- 1 tbsp balsamic vinegar

Directions:

1. Heat up a pan with the oil over medium heat, add the fish and cook for 5 mins on each side.
2. Add the rest of the ingredients, cook everything for 5 mins more, divide everything between plates and serve.

Nutrition:

- Calories 267
- Fat 11.2 g
- Carbs 1.5 g
- Protein 23 g

Parmesan Cod Mix

Prep Time: 10 mins

Servings: 4

Cooking: 11 mins

Ingredients:

- 1 tbsp lemon juice
- ½ cup chopped green onion
- 4 boneless cod fillets
- 3 minced garlic cloves
- 1 tbsp olive oil
- ½ cup shredded low-fat parmesan cheese

Directions:

1. Heat up a pan with the oil over medium heat, add the garlic and the green onions, toss and sauté for 5 mins.
2. Add the fish and cook it for 4 mins on each side.

3. Add the lemon juice, sprinkle the parmesan on top, cook everything for 2 mins more, divide between plates and serve.

Nutrition:

- Calories 275
- Fat 22.1 g
- Carbs 18.2 g
- Protein 12 g

Linguini with Clam Sauce

Prep Time: 10 mins

Servings: 4

Cooking: 11 mins

Ingredients:

- 12 oz whole-wheat linguini
- 1 tbsp olive oil
- 1 tbsp garlic, minced (about 2–3 cloves)
- 1 tbsp lemon juice
- 1 cup low-sodium chicken broth
- 2 cups canned whole clams, undrained
- 2 tbsp fresh parsley, minced (or 2 tsp dried)
- 1 tbsp butter

Directions:

1. In a 4-quart saucepan, bring 3 quarts of water to a boil over high heat.

2. Add linguini, and cook according to package directions for the shortest recommended time, about 9 mins.
3. Heat olive oil in a large saucepan. Add garlic, and cook gently until it begins to soften, about 30 seconds. Do not brown.
4. Add lemon juice and chicken broth. Bring to a boil.
5. Add clams, along with liquid, parsley, salt, pepper, and butter. Simmer just until heated through, about 1–2 mins. Do not overcook.
6. Strain the linguini, then add the pasta to the saucepan with the clams and mix well.
7. Divide into four equal portions (each about 2-1/2 cups), and serve.

Nutrition:
- Calories 476
- Fat 9 g
- Fiber 11 g
- Protein 34 g
- Carbs 66 g

Spicy Baked Fish

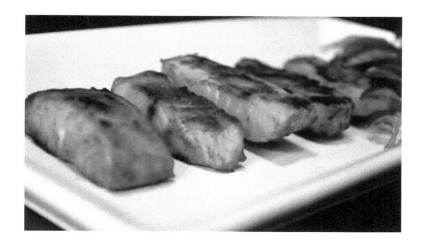

Prep Time: 5 mins

Servings: 5

Cooking: 15 mins

Ingredients:

- 1 tbsp olive oil
- 1 tsp. spice salt free seasoning
- 1 lb. salmon fillet

Directions:

1. Preheat the oven to 350F.
2. Sprinkle the fish with olive oil and the seasoning.
3. Bake for 15 min uncovered.
4. Slice and serve.

Nutrition:

- Calories 192
- Fat 11 g
- Carbs 14.9 g
- Protein 33.1 g

Smoked Trout Spread

Prep Time: 5 mins

Servings: 2

Ingredients:

- 2 tsps. Fresh lemon juice
- ½ cup low-fat cottage cheese
- 1 diced celery stalk
- ¼ lb. skinned smoked trout fillet,
- ½ tsp. Worcestershire sauce
- 1 tsp. hot pepper sauce
- ¼ cup coarsely chopped red onion

Directions:

1. Combine the trout, cottage cheese, red onion, lemon juice, hot pepper sauce and Worcestershire sauce in a blender or food processor.
2. Process until smooth, stopping to scrape down the sides of the bowl as needed.
3. Fold in the diced celery.

4. Keep in an air-tight container in the refrigerator.

Nutrition:

- Calories 57
- Fat 4 g
- Carbs 1 g
- Protein 4 g

Creamy Sea Bass Mix

Prep Time: 10 mins

Servings: 4

Cooking: 10 mins

Ingredients:

- 1 tbsp chopped parsley
- 2 tbsp avocado oil
- 1 cup coconut cream
- 1 tbsp lime juice
- 1 chopped yellow onion
- ¼ tsp. black pepper
- 4 boneless sea bass fillets

Directions:

1. Heat up a pan with the oil over medium heat, add the onion, toss and sauté for 2 mins.
2. Add the fish and cook it for 4 mins on each side.

3. Add the rest of the ingredients, cook everything for 4 mins more, divide between plates and serve.

Nutrition:

- Calories 283
- Fat 12.3 g
- Carbs 12.5 g
- Protein 8 g

Tuna Melt

Prep Time: 10 mins

Servings: 4

Ingredients:

- 3 oz. grated reduced-fat cheddar cheese
- 1/3 cup chopped celery
- Black pepper and salt
- ¼ cup chopped onion
- 2 whole-wheat English muffins
- 6 oz. drained white tuna
- ¼ cup low fat Russian

Directions:

1. Preheat broiler. Combine tuna, celery, onion and salad dressing.
2. Toast English muffin halves.
3. Place split-side-up on baking sheet and top each with 1/4 of tuna mixture.
4. Broil 2-3 mins or until heated through.

5. Top with cheese and return to broiler until cheese is melted, about 1 minute longer.

Nutrition:

- Calories 320
- Fat 16.7 g
- Carbs 17.1 g
- Protein 25.7 g

Crab Salad

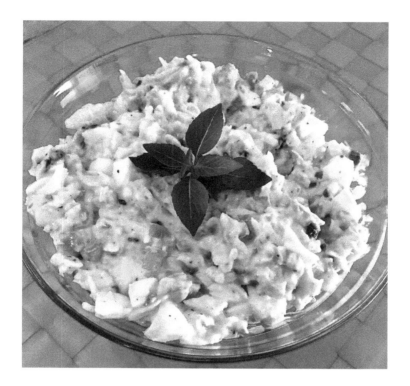

Prep Time: 10 mins

Servings: 4

Ingredients:

- 2 cup crab meat
- 1 cup halved cherry tomatoes

- 1 tbsp olive oil
- Black pepper
- 1 chopped shallot
- 1/3 cup chopped cilantro
- 1 tbsp lemon juice

Directions:

In a bowl, combine the crab with the tomatoes and the other ingredients; toss and serve.

Nutrition:

- Calories 54
- Fat 3.9 g
- Carbs 2.6 g
- Protein 2.3 g

Spicy Cod

Prep Time: 29 mins

Servings: 4

Cooking: 40 mins

Ingredients:

- 2 tbsp Fresh chopped parsley
- 2 lbs. cod fillets
- 2 cup low sodium salsa
- 1 tbsp flavorless oil

Directions:

1. Preheat the oven to 350°F.
2. In a large, deep baking dish drizzle the oil along the bottom. Place the cod fillets in the dish. Pour the salsa over the fish. Cover with foil for 20 mins. Remove the foil last 10 mins of cooking.
3. Bake in the oven for 20 – 30 mins, until the fish is flaky.

4. Serve with white or brown rice. Garnish with parsley.

Nutrition:

- Calories 110
- Fat 11 g
- Carbs 83 g
- Protein 16.5 g

Fish Tacos

Prep Time: 5 mins

Servings: 4

Cooking: 5 mins

Ingredients:

- 1 lb cod or white fish fillets, cut into 1-inch pieces
- 1 tbsp olive oil
- 2 tbsp lemon juice
- 1/2 package taco seasoning
- 12 (6-inch) warmed corn tortillas
- 1 cup shredded red cabbage
- 1 cup shredded green cabbage
- 2 cups chopped tomatoes
- 1/2 cup nonfat sour cream
- taco sauce to taste
- lime wedges for serving (optional)

Directions:

1. In a medium bowl, combine fish, olive oil, lemon juice, and seasoning mix; pour into a large skillet.
2. Cook, stirring constantly, over medium-high heat for 4 to 5 mins or until fish flakes easily when tested with a fork.
3. Fill tortillas with fish mixture.
4. Top with cabbage, tomato, sour cream, and taco sauce. Serve with lime wedge, if desired.

Nutrition:

- Calories 239
- Carbs 32 g
- Fiber 4 g
- Protein 19 g
- Fat 5 g

Lemony Scallop

Prep Time: 5 mins

Servings: 4

Cooking: 15 mins

Ingredients:

- 3 medium green peppers, cut into 1-1/2-inch squares
- 1-1/2 lbs fresh bay scallops
- 1 pint cherry tomatoes
- 1/4 cup dry white wine
- 1/4 cup vegetable oil
- 3 tbsp lemon juice
- dash garlic powder
- black pepper to taste

Directions:

1. Parboil green peppers for 2 mins.
2. Alternately thread first three ingredients on skewers.
3. Combine next five ingredients.

4. Brush kabobs with wine/oil/lemon mixture, place on grill (or under broiler).
5. Grill 15 mins, turning and basting frequently.

Nutrition:

- Calories 224
- Fat 6 g
- Carbs 83 g
- Protein 16.5 g

Baked Trout

Prep Time: 5 mins

Servings: 4

Cooking: 20 mins

Ingredients:

- 2 lbs trout fillet, cut into 6 pieces (any kind of fish can be used)
- 3 tbsp lime juice (about 2 limes)
- 1 medium tomato, chopped
- 1/2 medium onion, chopped
- 3 tbsp cilantro, chopped
- 1/2 tsp olive oil
- 1/4 tsp black pepper
- 1/4 tsp red pepper (optional)

Directions:

1. Preheat oven to 350F.
2. Rinse fish and pat dry. Place into baking dish.

3. In a separate dish, mix remaining ingredients together and pour over fish.
4. Bake for 15-20 mins or until fork-tender.

Nutrition:

- Calories 236

- Fat 9 g

- Protein 34 g

- Carbs 2 g

Shrimp Pasta Primavera

Prep Time: 15 mins

Servings: 6

Cooking: 15 mins

Ingredients:

- 1¼ cup sliced Asparagus
- 12 oz whole wheat Penne
- 1 cup Green peas
- 2 tsp Olive oil
- 1 tbsp minced Garlic
- 1/8 tsp crushed Red pepper
- 1 lb. Shrimp
- ½ cup sliced green onion
- 2 tsp Lemon juice
- 1 tbsp chopped Parsley
- 1/3 cup grated Parmesan cheese

Directions:

1. Set a large saucepan over high heat, and allow to come to a boil.
2. Once boiling, add asparagus then cook until fork tender (about 4 mins) Carefully remove the asparagus from the hot water using a slotted spoon then add your pasta to the same pot.
3. Cook until done based on the instructions on the package. When the pasta was 2 mins out add peas
4. When fully cooked, drain, and add to a large bowl with the asparagus
5. Set a skillet with olive oil over medium heat, then add red pepper, and garlic, then cook, while stirring for about a minute
6. Add shrimp and cook until it becomes opaque (about 4 mins), stirring
7. Add your remaining Ingredients: to the skillet on top of shrimp and toss to coat.

Nutrition:

- Calories 440
- Protein 31g
- Carbs 31g
- Fat 18g

Brown Stewed Fish

Prep Time: 10 mins

Servings: 4

Cooking: 10 mins

Ingredients:

- 2 lbs fish
- 1 diced large onion
- 2 small tomatoes
- 3 stalks scallion
- 1 cup Vegetables
- ¾ cup fish stock
- 2 slices hot pepper
- ¼ cup oil

Directions:

1. Scale, clean and prepare fish for frying

2. Allow oil to cool, strain nearly all of it from frying pan, put aside Sauté seasonings and vegetables in frying pan

3. Add water or stock to frying pan with sautéed vegetables and simmer until all flavors blend

4. Add fish, cover and cook for five mins.

Nutrition:

- Calories 352
- Protein 36g
- Carbs 14g
- Fat 17g

Grilled Cod

Prep Time: 15 mins

Servings: 2

Cooking: 15 mins

Ingredients:

- 2 cod fillets
- ½ tsp garlic paste
- 3 tbsp lemon juice
- ½ tsp black pepper
- ½ tsp oregano
- 1 tsp fish sauce
- ¼ tsp turmeric powder
- 2 tbsp olive oil

Directions:

1. Sprinkle turmeric powder on fish and rub all over
2. Leave it for 10-15 mins then wash out fish well

3. Take a bowl add vinegar, lemon juice, pepper, salt, fish sauce and oregano, toss to combine

4. Spread this mixture on fish fillets and rub on it with hands

Nutrition:

- Calories 138
- Protein 271g
- Carbs 46g
- Fat 7g

Baked Salmon

Prep Time: 10 mins

Servings: 6

Cooking: 10 mins

Ingredients:

- 1½ lbs salmon fillets
- ½ sliced onion
- 1 cup chopped grape tomatoes
- 1 tsp dried basil
- 1 tbsp chopped chives
- 1 tsp dried rosemary
- 1 tsp garlic powder
- 1/3 cup soy sauce
- 1/3 cup brown sugar
- 1/3 cup Water
- ¼ cup vegetable oil

Directions:

1. Preheat oven to 350° F
2. Season salmon fillets with onion, basil, rosemary, garlic powder, and salt
3. Combine brown sugar, soy sauce, water, and vegetable oil until sugar is dissolved
4. Place fillets in a Ziploc bag or airtight container with soy sauce mixture and place in refrigerator for 2 hours to marinate
5. Preheat grill at medium heat. Lightly oil grill grate. Place fillets on the preheated grill and cook for 6 to 8 mins per side.

Nutrition:

- Calories: 274
- Protein 24g
- Carbs 1g
- Fat 19g

Steamed Mussels

Prep Time: 5 mins

Servings: 4

Cooking: 10 mins

Ingredients:

- 6 oz chorizo
- 1 cup white wine
- 2 tbsp olive oil
- 1 sliced onion
- 4 lbs Mussels
- 3 sprigs thyme
- 1 tsp smoked paprika
- 15 oz diced tomatoes
- 4 sliced garlic cloves

Directions:

1. over medium heat, warm olive oil

2. Add the onion, season to taste and cook until softened for 3-4 mins
3. Add garlic and cook for an additional 1 minute
4. Stir in the smoked paprika and cook for 30 seconds or until fragrant
5. Add the chorizo, wine, and tomatoes
6. Add the fresh thyme and bring to a simmer
7. Stir in the mussels and coat with sauce
8. Cover and cook until mussels are opened
9. Discard all unopened ones
10. Serve mussels while still hot with toasted bread slices.

Nutrition:

- Calories 256
- Protein 34g
- Carbs 198g

Creamy Seafood and Veggies Soup

Prep Time: 10 mins

Servings: 12

Cooking: 3 hours

Ingredients:

- 10 oz coconut cream
- 2 cups low-sodium veggie stock
- 2 cups no-salt-added tomato sauce
- 12 oz canned crab meat, no-salt-added and drained
- 1 and ½ cups water
- 1 and ½ lbs jumbo shrimp, peeled and deveined
- 1 yellow onion, chopped
- 1 cup carrots, chopped
- 4 tilapia fillets, skinless, boneless and cubed
- 2 celery stalks, chopped
- 3 kale stalks, chopped
- 1 bay leaf
- 2 garlic cloves, minced

- ½ tsp cloves, ground
- 1 tsp rosemary, dried
- 1 tsp thyme, dried

Directions:

1. In your slow cooker, mix coconut cream with stock, tomato sauce and water and stir.
2. Add shrimp, fish, onion, carrots, celery, kale, garlic, bay leaf, cloves, thyme and rosemary, cover, cook on Low for 3 hours, stir, ladle into bowls and serve.

Nutrition:

- Calories 220
- Fat 3g
- Fiber 3g
- Carbs 8g
- Protein 7g

Seafood Gumbo

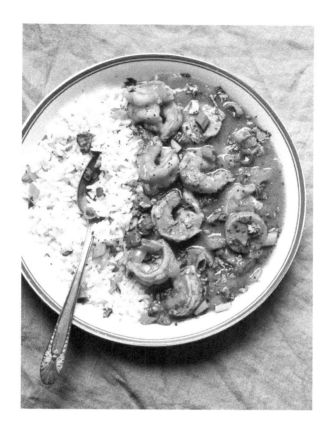

Prep Time: 10 mins

Servings: 4

Cooking: 6 hours

Ingredients:

- 1 lb shrimp, peeled and deveined
- 2 lbs mussels, cleaned and debearded
- 28 oz canned clams, no-salt-added and drained
- 1 yellow onion, chopped
- 10 oz canned tomato paste, no-salt-added

Directions:

In your slow cooker, mix shrimp with mussels, clams, onion and tomato paste, stir, cover, cook on Low for 6 hours, divide into bowls and serve.

Nutrition:

- Calories 200
- Fat 3g
- Fiber 2g
- Carbs 7g
- Protein 5g

Lemon and Spinach Trout

Prep Time: 10 mins

Servings: 4

Cooking: 2 hours

Ingredients:

- 2 lemons, sliced
- ¼ cup low sodium chicken stock
- 2 tbsp dill, chopped
- 12 oz spinach
- 4 medium trout

Directions:

1. Put the stock in your slow cooker and add the fish inside
2. Season with black pepper to the taste, top with lemon slices, dill and spinach, cover and cook on High for 2 hours.

3. Divide fish, lemon and spinach between plates and serve

Nutrition:

- Calories 240
- Fat 5g
- Fiber 4g
- Carbs 9g
- Protein 14g

Easy Roast Salmon with Roasted Asparagus

Prep Time: 5 mins

Servings: 4

Cooking: 15 mins

Ingredients:

- 2 (5-ounce) salmon fillets with skin
- 2 tsps olive oil, plus extra for drizzling
- 1 bunch asparagus, trimmed
- 1 tsp dried chives
- 1 tsp dried tarragon
- Fresh lemon wedges for serving

Directions:

1. Preheat the oven to 425°F.
2. Rub salmon completely with 1 tsp of olive oil per fillet. Season with salt and pepper.

3. Place asparagus spears on a foil lined baking sheet and lay the salmon fillets skin-side down on top. Put pan in upper-third of oven and roast until fish is just cooked through (about 12 mins). Roasting time will vary depending on the thickness of your salmon. Salmon should flake easily with a fork when it's ready and an instant-read thermometer should register 145°F.
4. When cooked, remove from the oven, cut fillets in half crosswise, then lift flesh from skin with a metal spatula and transfer to a plate.
5. Discard the skin. Drizzle salmon with oil, sprinkle with herbs, and serve with lemon wedges and roasted asparagus spears.

Nutrition:

- Calories 220
- Fat 3g
- Fiber 3g
- Carbs 8g
- Protein 7g

Shrimp Pasta Primavera

Prep Time: 5 mins

Servings: 2

Cooking: 15 mins

Ingredients:

- 2 tbsp olive oil
- 1 tbsp garlic, minced
- 2 cups assorted fresh vegetables, chopped coarsely (zucchini, broccoli, asparagus or whatever you prefer)
- 4 oz frozen shrimp, cooked, peeled, and deveined
- Freshly ground black pepper
- Juice of ½ lemon
- 4 oz whole-wheat angel-hair pasta, cooked per package instructions
- 2 tbsp grated Parmesan cheese

Directions:

1. Heat the oil in a large nonstick skillet over medium heat. Add the garlic and sauté for 1 minute.
2. Add vegetables and sauté until crisp tender (about 3 to 4 mins)
3. Add the shrimp and sauté until just heated through. Season lightly with salt and pepper and squeeze lemon juice over the shrimp and vegetables. Continue to cook for about 2 mins until the juices have been reduced by about half. Remove from heat
4. Toss shrimp and vegetables with pasta. Serve topped with Parmesan cheese

Nutrition:

- Calories 439
- Fat 17g
- Carbs 50g
- Fiber 8g
- Protein 23g

Cilantro-Lime Tilapia Tacos

Prep Time: 10 mins

Servings: 4

Cooking: 10 mins

Ingredients:

- 1 tsp olive oil
- 1 lb tilapia fillets, rinsed and dried
- 3 cups diced tomatoes
- ½ cup fresh cilantro, chopped, plus additional for serving
- 3 tbsp freshly squeezed lime juice
- Freshly ground black pepper
- 8 (5-inch) white-corn tortillas
- 1 avocado sliced into 8 wedges
- Optional: lime wedges and fat-free sour cream for serving

Directions:

1. Heat the oil in a large skillet, add the tilapia and Cook until the flesh starts to flake (about 5 mins per side).
2. Add the tomatoes, cilantro, and lime juice. Sauté over medium-high heat for about 5 mins, breaking up the fish and mixing well
3. Heat tortillas in a skillet for a few mins on each side to warm.
4. Serve ¼ cup of fish mixture on each warmed tortilla with two slices of avocado.
5. Serve immediately with optional toppings.

Nutrition:

- Calories 286
- Fat 12g
- Carbs 22g
- Fiber 4g
- Protein 28g

Garlic and Butter Sword Fish

Prep Time: 10 mins

Servings: 4

Cooking: 2 hours and 30 mins

Ingredients:

- ½ cup melted butter
- 6 chopped garlic cloves
- 1 tbsp black pepper
- 5 sword fish fillets

Directions:

1. Take a mixing bowl and toss in all of your garlic, black pepper alongside the melted butter
2. Take a parchment paper and place your fish fillet in that paper
3. Cover it up with the butter mixture and wrap up the fish

4. Repeat the process until all of your fish are wrapped up
5. Let it cook for 2 and a half hours and release the pressure naturally
6. Serve

Nutrition:

- Calories 379
- Fat 26 g
- Carbs 1 g
- Protein 34 g

Pressure Cooker Crab Legs

Prep Time: 5 mins

Servings: 4

Cooking: 17 mins

Ingredients:

- 1 sliced lemon piece
- 1 cup water
- 1 cup melted butter
- 2 lbs. crab legs
- 1 cup white wine

Directions:

1. Add water to your Instant Pot alongside wine
2. Add crab legs
3. Lock up the lid and cook on HIGH pressure for 7 mins
4. Release the pressure naturally over 10 mins
5. Open the lid and add melted butter and a dash of lemon

6. Enjoy

Nutrition:

- Calories 191
- Fat 1 g
- Carbs 0 g
- Protein 41 g

Delicious Tuna Sandwich

Prep Time: 15 mins

Servings: 2

Cooking: 17 mins

Ingredients:

- 30 g olive oil
- 1 peeled and diced medium cucumber
- 2 ½ g pepper
- 4 whole wheat bread slices
- 85 g diced onion
- 1 can flavored tuna
- 85 g shredded spinach

Directions:

1. Grab your blender and add the spinach, tuna, onion, oil, salt and pepper in, and pulse for about 10 to 20 seconds.

2. In the meantime, toast your bread and add your diced cucumber to a bowl, which you can pour your tuna mixture in. Carefully mix and add the mixture to the bread once toasted.
3. Slice in half and serve, while storing the remaining mixture in the fridge.

Nutrition:

- Calories 302
- Fat 5.8 g
- Carbs 36.62 g
- Protein 28 g

Easy Mussels

Prep Time: 10 mins

Servings: 4

Cooking: 17 mins

Ingredients:

- 2 lbs. cleaned mussels
- 4 minced garlic cloves
- 2 chopped shallots
- Lemon and parsley
- 2 tbsp Butter
- ½ cup broth
- ½ cup white wine

Directions:

1. Clean the mussels and remove the beard
2. Discard any mussels that do not close when tapped against a hard surface

3. Set your pot to Sauté mode and add chopped onion and butter
4. Stir and sauté onions
5. Add garlic and cook for 1 minute
6. Add broth and wine
7. Lock up the lid and cook for 5 mins on HIGH pressure
8. Release the pressure naturally over 10 mins
9. Serve with a sprinkle of parsley and enjoy!

Nutrition:

- Calories 286
- Fat 14 g
- Carbs 12 g
- Protein 28 g

Parmesan-Crusted Fish

Prep Time: 5 mins

Servings: 4

Cooking: 7-8 mins

Ingredients:

- ¾ tsp. ground ginger
- 1/3 cup panko bread crumbs
- Mixed fresh salad greens
- ¼ cup finely shredded parmesan cheese
- 1 tbsp butter
- 4 skinless cod fillets
- 3 cup julienned carrots

Directions:

1. Preheat oven to 450° F. Lightly coat a baking sheet with nonstick cooking spray.
2. Rinse and pat dry fish; place on baking sheet. Season with salt and pepper.

3. In small bowl stir together crumbs and cheese; sprinkle on fish.
4. Bake, uncovered, 4 to 6 mins for each 1/2-inch thickness of fish, until crumbs are golden and fish flakes easily when tested with a fork.
5. Meanwhile, in a large skillet bring 1/2 cup water to boiling; add carrots. Reduce heat.
6. Cook, covered, for 5 mins. Uncover; cook 2 mins more. Add butter and ginger; toss.
7. Serve fish and carrots with greens.

Nutrition:

- Calories 216.4
- Fat 10.1 g
- Carbs 1.3 g
- Protein 29.0 g

Salmon and Horseradish Sauce

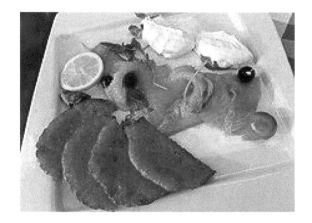

Prep Time: 10 mins

Servings: 4

Cooking: 7 mins

Ingredients:

- ½ cup coconut cream
- 1 tbsp Prepared horseradish
- 4 de-boned medium salmon fillets
- 2 tbsp Chopped dill

- 1 ½ tbsp Organic olive oil
- ¼ tsp. black pepper

Directions:

1. Heat up a pan while using the oil over medium-high heat, add salmon fillets, season with black pepper and cook for 5 mins one each side.
2. In a bowl, combine the cream with the dill and horseradish and whisk well.
3. Divide the salmon between plates and serve with all the horseradish cream for the top.

Nutrition:

- Calories 275
- Fat12 g
- Carbs 14 g
- Protein 27 g

Crunchy Topped Fish with Potato Sticks

Prep Time: 5 mins

Servings: 4

Cooking: 7 mins

Ingredients:

- 2 tbsp Melted margarine
- Nonstick spray coating
- ¾ cup crushed herb-seasoned stuffing mix
- 12 oz. sliced medium baking potatoes
- 2 tsps. Melted cooking oil
- 16 oz. fresh catfish fillets
- Garlic salt

Directions:

1. Rinse fish and pat dry with paper towels; set aside.
2. Line a large baking sheet with foil. Spray foil with nonstick spray coating.

3. Arrange potato sticks in a single layer over half of the baking sheet. Brush potatoes with oil or the 2 tsps melted margarine. Sprinkle with garlic salt.
4. Bake in a 450 degree F oven for 10 mins.
5. Meanwhile, stir together stuffing mix and the 2 tbsps melted margarine.
6. Place fish on baking sheet next to potatoes. Sprinkle stuffing mix over fish. Return pan to oven and bake 9 to 12 mins more or until fish flakes easily when tested with a fork and potatoes are tender.

Nutrition:

- Calories 94
- Fat 6.19g
- Carbs 9.6 g
- Protein 1.2 g

Halibut and Cherry Tomatoes

Prep Time: 10 mins

Servings: 4

Cooking: 8 mins

Ingredients:

- 3 minced garlic cloves
- 4 skinless halibut fillets
- 2 cup cherry tomatoes
- 2 tbsp Chopped basil
- ¼ tsp. black pepper
- 1 ½ tbsp Organic olive oil
- 2 tbsp Balsamic vinegar

Directions:

1. Heat up a pan with 1 tbsp organic essential olive oil, add halibut fillets, cook them for 5 mins on both sides and divide between plates.

2. Heat up another pan because of the rest within the oil over medium-high heat, add the tomatoes, garlic, vinegar and basil, toss, cook for 3 mins, add next on the fish and serve.

Nutrition:

- Calories 221
- Fat 4 g
- Carbs 6 g
- Protein 21 g

Salmon and Cauliflower Mix

Prep Time: 10 mins

Servings: 4

Cooking: 20 mins

Ingredients:

- 4 boneless salmon fillets
- 2 tbsp Coconut aminos
- 1 sliced big red onion
- ¼ cup coconut sugar
- 1 head separated cauliflower florets
- 2 tbsp Olive oil

Directions:

1. In a smaller bowl, mix sugar with coconut aminos and whisk.
2. Heat up a pan with half the oil over medium-high heat, add cauliflower and onion, stir and cook for 10 mins.

3. Put the salmon inside baking dish, drizzle the remainder inside oil, add coconut aminos, toss somewhat, season with black pepper, introduce within the oven and bake at 400 º F for 10 mins.
4. Divide the salmon along using the cauliflower mix between plates and serve.

Nutrition:

- Calories 220
- Fat 3 g
- Carbs 12 g
- Protein 9 g

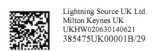

Lightning Source UK Ltd.
Milton Keynes UK
UKHW020630140621
385475UK00001B/29